Joyful Warrior

JOYFUL WARRIOR

A GUIDE TO OVERCOME ANXIETY AND
UPLIFT YOUR MOOD

KEIANA PHILLIPS

SELF-PUBLISHED

DEDICATION

This book is dedicated to all of my warriors out there, fighting each day to chase their dreams, protect their peace, and live joyfully especially in hard circumstances. In seasons that make you want to give up, or run the other way!

But you FIGHT! You keep pressing forward, despite it all.
This book is for YOU my sweet, strong friend.
My fellow Joyful Warriors the victory is ours!

EPIGRAPH

"Let me take a moment to tell those of you who are dealing with and fighting through something painful: it is a miracle that you're sitting here. You are nobly doing your best to battle your way through it. You are a warrior because of the trials you are going through, but don't you dare squander the strength you have earned just because the acquisition of it was painful."

Taken from Girl, Wash Your Face by Rachel Hollis
© 2018 by Rachel Hollis
Used by permission of Thomas Nelson.
www.thomasnelson.com

Contents

FORWARD

This guide is a wealth of knowledge! Over the years Keiana's coaching has been such an asset to my well-being and overall outlook; her guidance on business, life, and motherhood is tried and true. Her collection of the best tips from top motivational speakers makes it easy for clients to enjoy the relevant parts without needing to do any of the digging themselves. A great stand alone item for staying healthy during the pandemic, or you can include the product recommendations and tangible tips into a new routine, and implement them into your life immediately!

-Claire Bussell, // Owner www.claireb3d.com

It's been an amazing couple of years as I have learned so much from my dear sister in Christ, Keiana Phillips. We met through a mutual friend and connected immediately. We've shared business successes and failures, frustrations, as well as exhilarating moments. Keiana and I created a business affiliation and cultivated a love for all things holistic.

I own an all-natural skin care and wellness company. My husband and I grow many of our own herbs, flowers, plants and fruits on our farm, which we use in the formulation of our products. Keiana fell in love with my essential oils and has really enjoyed incorporating these ancient biblical oils in her holistic approach of helping her body heal from anxiety. The power of essential oils dates back thousands of years. The Egyptians, Romans, and other ancient cultures used them for healing everything from common ailments and to protect the mind from anxiety and adrenal fatigue.

The truth is, I've probably learned equally as much from Keiana as she has learned from me. I watch her as she works so hard to balance her family life, being a young mother; all the while combating, on a daily basis, the crippling anxiety that can hit her like a mack truck. I'm so proud of her emotional growth and the spiritual beauty that arises from her soul. This book will touch so many at the core and help those who feel so alone in their battle with anxiety.

-Regina Azarte, // Owner www.trinity-fit.com

INTRODUCTION

I believe as we walk through life we will face all kinds of seasons, whether it be amazing, good, comfortable, contentment or a raging storm, in addition to the four seasons of the calendar year. Unexpected curve balls will come our way and can change our season of life from amazing to dreadful. How am I going to feel on the other side of this? How am I going to manage through this? Should I have done more two months ago? Rest assured friend, you're not alone. The struggle in adulting just got too real way too fast. Which is why it's more important now, than ever, that we stick together.

It was only three months ago we jumped into this new year with an amazing word of the year, new planner and left all the baggage from 2019 in the past – totally ready to crush 2020! Whether you had plans to focus on your walk with God more, get through a few personal development books, gratitude journaling or to overall be a kinder human.

Somewhere along the way in the days, weeks and months you fall right back into where you were the year before. Only difference is by this time of the year you begin to lose hope because of unforeseen circumstances taht make you feel isolated in a situation that you can't control.

Not that long ago agoraphobia forced me into my own isolation, during various seasons in my life. So, in a season where I can get in my car without the fear of a panic attack, and drive to places that I once upon a time couldn't, like the mall or beach; I now can't. This is all overwhelming and rather annoying. It's still supposed to be that new year vibe where we're focusing on being positive but then THIS. How do I stay positive without letting anxiety creep back or bouts of depression when I can't do the normal activities I've adopted, to improve my physical, mental and emotional health?

Grab a cup of coffee and let's figure this out together. My hope is that sharing a little bit about my own journey, as well as some practical tips, tools and resources will help us walk through this crazy surreal moment in time, and come out thriving on the other side!

DISCLAIMER

This book is not intended as a substitute for the medical advice of physicians. The reader should regularly consult a physician in matters relating to his/her health and particularly with respect to any symptoms that may require diagnosis or medical attention.

|| IMPORTANT ||

If you or anyone you know are struggling with suicidal ideation please seek help immediately. You are not alone.
The National Suicide Prevention Lifeline is:
800-273-8255
Website: https://suicidepreventionlifeline.org

DON'T LET ISOLATION STEAL YOUR JOY

Isolation is an uncomfortable season of life to be in, it's lonely and unpredictable. How incredibly boring would life be, what lessons would we learn, what growth would we have gained if we knew exactly the moment a hard season would show up? We'd prepare for it and not grow from it. Times that test our faith, challenges our strength and pushes us towards a better version of ourselves, are where our greatest victories will come.

In my own experience being stuck inside (literally) is hard, especially when all you want to do is get out in the fresh air, jump in your car and go. For me, it did lead into a depression, which ultimately made the anxiety even worse. It can make you feel as though you are on this vicious cycle with no way of escape. However, let me tell you there is definitely light at the end of the tunnel. Storms don't last forever, right? Seasons come and seasons go.

My first piece of advice is to give yourself the grace you need to feel all of the emotions you're going through. At the end of the day we have all had to adjust our lives with little warning; and it kind of sucks. Whether you feel angry, sad, scared, annoyed or whatever. It's okay! We are all in the same boat, even if it's a totally different season for you. My second piece of advice is you can either use a difficult time to avoid dealing with the reality by binge watching shows (been there, watched the entire season of Gilmore Girls and Gossip Girl) or use this time to begin working on you, whether that's spiritually, physically, or focusing on a new hobby. We are so blessed that even in a time of isolation we have technology, which gives us access to so many tools to enrich our lives from the comfort of our own homes. Use them!!! You are not alone. Get an accountability partner who you trust to walk alongside you in this journey. Please reach out to me and I will add you to my personal accountability group that I run. My third piece of advice that I will cover throughout this guide is how to focus on your overall mental health, good nutrition, as well as fitness, which are all vital in maintaining a positive healthy mindset.

TAKE ACTION NOW!

1. Meditate. I used to think mediation was such a weird concept. Even the bible tells us to meditate on his word, day and night. Yet, I somehow just didn't comprehend in general what it meant until I developed a love for personal development books. Our minds are working nonstop with thought after thought, task after task, which tends to increase anxiety. We need to take moments out of our day to either meditate on God's word, prayer, take a moment to be still and thankful, or turn on an uplifting podcast/audio book.

YOUR MENTAL HEALTH MATTERS

Mind you, mental and emotional well-being, as a Christian woman, has more of a stigma than out there in the world. I lived in fear for a long time to get the help I needed. I refused to take medication for months because of the shame I felt inside. How do you deal with the gut wrenching struggles in these areas, whether you're a Christian woman, mom, student, working woman or boss? No matter where you are on the spectrum, at one time or another you have had to come to terms that at some point you are not okay. You find yourself in an overwhelming state of constant anxiety. You will do anything humanly possible to avoid having to talk about the deep dark internal battles causing the anxiety, which just won't seem to go away no matter how hard you try.

Let me touch on a little bit about my own journey, with not just depression but more so anxiety, and what it looked like for me. (You will be able to learn more about my walk through this on my blog coming soon to my website) Anxiety is a normal part of life, whether it's a flutter of butterflies in your stomach as you're getting ready for your wedding day, or that "I may puke " before a big presentation. These feelings are circumstantial and once it's over they go away. No, the anxiety I am speaking of is being in an ongoing state of worry or fear that leads your body to automatically go into flight or fight, which if not combatted immediately will turn into a full blown panic attack. I have had to struggle with debilitating panic attacks for years, to the point where I couldn't leave the house and never thought it would end. It's the cycle of anxiety leading to panic attacks that then eventually threw me into a season of full-blown agoraphobia. Mind you I had no idea what this was until I found a therapist that specializes in panic disorder. It was then that I started to have a better understanding of what was happening to me.

Excerpt From: Think Learn Succeed

"When you express your emotions in a healthy way, you allow the free flow of neuropeptides and energy, which allows all bodily systems to function as a healthy whole. However, when you repress and deny your emotions, whatever they may be, you block the network of quantum and chemical pathways, stopping the flow of good chemicals that run your biology and behavior. You will be working against your customized, wired-for-love mode. When you do this for years, you are essentially becoming expert at not feeling what you feel, which in turn creates tremendous conflict in your mind and damage in your brain.

Unfortunately, many of us have become experts at hiding our emotions—or think we have. Instead we create neurochemical chaos in our brains. Signs of suppressed feelings arising from this conflict include irritability, short temper, overreactivity, anxiety, frustration, fear, impulsiveness, a desire for control, perfectionism, and self-doubt."

Taken from Think, Learn, Succeed by Dr. Caroline Leaf
© 2018 by Caroline Leaf
Used by permission from the author. www.drleaf.com

Guess what though? No matter where you

are mentally or emotionally you are not defined by it. You are not defined by the lies people have spoken over you, the labels the doctors have given you or the medication you are taking. You are a child of God. A gift to the world. You matter. Every single part of you matters, especially your heart. You are meant for so much more than you have given yourself credit for. There is hope on the other side even if it doesn't feel like it today. You have to decide if you're willing to fight for that joy, peace and happiness. Are you willing to fight with me, friend?

Take Action Now!

1. Start learning deep-breathing exercises. Learning to do this will change your life forever!!!! If you have an Apple watch, or any kind of tracker, there should be a breathing tool built in as a reminder to help you pause a moment to breathe and/or regulate your breathing. YouTube is also a great source for videos on how to properly learn the skill of deep breathing.

2. Start a gratitude journal. This is one of those things you hear all the motivational speakers talk about that seems cheesy, right? Let me assure you there is nothing better to help you improve your

mood, thoughts, and shift your mindset than starting your day focusing on the things you're grateful for.

3. Lavender. Lavender. Lavender. I can't emphasize enough the incredible benefits of a pure therapeutic grade lavender essential oil. I literally use lavender daily, I put dabs behind my ears, mix with my lotion and diffuse. It helps calm your mood almost instantly just by the beautiful aroma.

4. A disclaimer is most definitely needed for this one...Before my fellow believers close the book here. I'd like to cultivate a space for keeping an open mind for holistic wellness. Full Spectrum Hemp, or CBD, which is simply one component of many from the hemp plant. I have become knowledgeable in this area over the last couple of years. I've been privileged to see doctors speak on the topic, as well as industry leaders. Let me first start by saying do your research... I promise it's worth it!!! I'm not going to lie, I thought any hemp product would get you high, until I got educated and started taking full spectrum hemp oil daily. It increased my mood, energy and got rid of the headaches I struggled with all the time.

The hemp plant is NOT the same as the marijuana

plant, again not the same although they're in the same family of cannabis. Marijuana contains high amounts of THC (tetrahydrocannabinol) which give you the psychoactive (high) feeling. Hemp/CBD contains virtually no THC while having all the benefits such as mental calmness, reduces anxiety, natural sleep-aid, anti-inflammatory and improves your overall health and wellness -non-addictive**. These are just a handful of benefits. In the resource section in the back I have links to great informative articles.

KALE SALAD PLEASE

Just kidding, I personally am not a fan of kale salads. I am, however, going to talk a bit about *drum roll...* NUTRITION! Oh my how isolation, anxiety and being overwhelmed can lead to the worst food decisions. Sweet tooth junkie here! When you're stressed out the last thing on your mind is to reach for carrots with a perfectly portioned amount of ranch. Nope! You're going for that chocolate cupcake or donut. This isn't about a diet, this is about a lifestyle – no matter what season of life you're in. What you put in your body has a deep impact on your brain, and of course, your health in general.

In my darkest moments I have battled with

anorexia, I would go from obsessively counting calories, to not caring about anything and consuming mass amounts of sugar. When I got pregnant I was extremely underweight for my height and age. As my body began to change during pregnancy it was hard to watch the scale move up, I didn't think I'd ever lose the baby weight. So, I've struggled with numerous body image issues. I've seen first hand how bad eating habits and poor nutrition can cause your body to be out of alignment, which in turn affects your brain while keeping you in a pattern of continuing to make poor food decisions. Although, it may feel good for a moment, that regret will always creep in. You want to do better, eat better, exercise etc., yet you use your current circumstance to justify staying exactly where you are; making decisions you know are so bad for your health. The road isn't easy my friend, trust me! But, if I can dig myself out of the bad nutrition pit, I believe you can be too lovely – you're worth it.

Excerpt From: Think & Eat Yourself Smart
"Research shows that 75–98 percent of current mental, physical, emotional, and behavioral illnesses and issues come from our thought life; only 2–25 percent come from a combination of genetics and what enters our bodies

through food, medications, pollution, chemicals, and so on.1 These statistics show that the mindset behind the meal—the thinking behind the meal—plays a dominant role in the process of human food-related health issues, approximately 80 percent. Hence the title of this book: you have to think and eat yourself smart, happy, and healthy.

If we do not have a healthy mind, then nothing else in our life will be healthy, including our eating habits."

Taken from Think & Eat Yourself Smart by Dr. Caroline Leaf
© 2016 by Caroline Leaf
Used by permission from the author. www.drleaf.com

Good nutrition honestly isn't about depriving yourself of the things you love. It's about having the things you love in moderation and loving the good nutrition that fuels your body, mind and soul. That being said, this isn't something that will just happen overnight. You have to first make the decision to eat better, then turn those choices into healthy habits – which takes time like everything else in life. There's no magic pill, If there was I'd be first in line-ha. You have to put in the work in order to get the results you want.

Take Action Now!

1. H2O!!!! Staying hydrated is so important. As a mom, sometimes I forget to slow down and drink water. We are to drink half our weight in ounces (so if you weigh 140 pounds you should be drinking 70 ounces daily). In order for me to keep track I either buy a 50oz pre-filled water bottle, or I keep my own bottle with ounces listed on the side so I can keep track of my water intake daily. If you are not hydrated enough it can affect the way your brain functions, which will only increase your anxiety more. Our blood is more than 90% of water, so it's vital that we keep ourselves hydrated daily. A good way to start is/the transition first to sparkling water or add slices of lemon or lime to water, which adds alkaline as a bonus!

2. Cut back on sugar, caffeine, soda and the foods from the middle aisles. This will be challenging – oh, I can't begin to tell you. I actually had to STOP drinking coffee cold turkey, headaches and all for over 2 years, but it was just making my anxiety worse. Sugar and junk food is a no brainer, we all know it's not healthy for us, but how easy we cave in to it's delicious ways. But, here's some good news, you don't need to give it up completely! You have to

be realistic with yourself. Set small goals to cut back, and as you do, you'll start to see how amazing you will feel again. I'll be honest, now that my anxiety is better I do drink lattes now, but my compromise is I don't keep coffee in my home so I don't go down the path of consuming multiple cups a day, like in the past. Find a trick that works well for you to cut back, and you'll find the shift will come more easily.

3. Supplementation is really important to me. I've learned over the years that you can have the healthiest diet but still lack important micronutrients, vitamins and minerals. Research has shown the depletion of soil quality over the years has stripped away a lot of those nutrients we used to be able to get from our fruits and vegetables. This is why it's important to also stay on top of your annual physicals, so you can know where to supplement in one area and not to overdo it in another. My favorite kinds of supplements aren't the ones you find from your local store. I like to be sure there is some sort of research or science supporting the supplement and/ or company. I have listed a few in the back in the Warrior Directory!

4. If you would like the help of a coach to walk alongside you in your nutrition journey. I am a

certified nutrition coach and I provide online nutrition coaching. If you would like more information on my nutrition coaching services please email me at info@joyfulwarriorbook.com. I would love to work with you!

THAT GOOD HURT

I am talking about that pain you feel when you're trying to pee but you can barely sit because it hurts so bad from the workout you did the day before. That's the good kind of hurt I'm talking about. The pain that is uncomfortable, but a reminder that you worked hard. Even though you can't see the results yet, with consistency you will hit the goal that you are shooting for.

When I was in the midst of postpartum depression, and then experienced an extremely traumatic event when my son was about a year and a half, I started to struggle with suicidal thoughts. I had honestly turned my back on God. My anxiety was beginning to climb, and to top it off I was completely mortified with my body. I hated how I looked while I was also feeling empty on the inside. I knew what I needed to get back to a consistent workout regime but couldn't seem to get it together. Again, shame consumed me.

Excerpt From: #MAXOUT Your Life
"I believe it's of the utmost importance to take care of our physical body. It provides us the energy, confidence and strength we need to win in business and in life. When we're fit, healthy and active we feel our best. Feeling good is important because our body is the temple of our soul and our mind, which is the source of our strength and power.

Keeping a healthy physical routine is one more way you are keeping a promise to yourself. It's a daily validation that you are worthy and value yourself to keep your promises to you."

Taken from #MAXOUT Your Life by Ed Mylett
© 2018 by Ed Mylett
Used by permission from the author. www.edmylett.com

Working out does increase your happiness as it releases that wonderful chemical called endorphins as well as serotonin. The problem is you have to get there consistently. Just like with your nutrition, your fitness has to become a habit, which isn't created overnight. For me, it took taking small steps with my nutrition and fitness, to get to a place where my mental health started to improve. Once you can find a favorite type of fitness, it'll be easier to stick to it, and you'll find yourself falling in love with working out – I promise. For me, personally, it's lifting weights and building lean toned muscles. Yes, ladies, lifting weights are good for us because strength training burns fat especially on your belly, booty and arms! Your fitness journey in particular I believe your fitness journey is the hardest one. It's easy to always make an excuse not to workout or hit the gym – guilty!!! This is your marathon my friend, not a race. If you stumble, pick yourself up and keep going.

TAKE ACTION NOW!

1. Sleep...zzz! The amount of sleep you get daily will also have a great impact on your anxiety levels. Plus, your body needs it to heal and recover. If you're a mom, like me, sleep is so precious once your kid(s) get to a sleeping age. The less sleep I get, the more irritable and anxious I am. Really, listen to your

body, take a nap if you need to. Sleep with your phone away from you so you aren't distracted right before bed. I like to listen to meditations at night to help calm my mind, which help me fall into a deep sleep faster. I will include some great meditation apps in the back resources section.

2. Take a stroll. To get started on your fitness journey, try incorporating a 15-30min walk into your schedule daily. Walking has been proven to improve your mood, it's known to strengthen your heart, and can also increase your immune system and energy. The best part is you can do this for free! You may even turn walking into a love of running. You'll never know until you try.

3. If you would like help getting started on your fitness journey please reach out to me at info@joyfulwarriorbook.com.

THIS ISN'T THE END, IT'S THE BEGINNING

When my anxiety was at its worst, the panic attacks kept me isolated. I would pray and ask God to just take me home. Anything would be better than this personal hell I was in. Honestly, I didn't want to die, I wanted to live again. I wanted my life back so badly. But, I couldn't see the light at the end of the tunnel all I felt was the agony of being trapped.

As I've walked through this journey I've realized how thankful I am for it. It wasn't just the anxiety I've had to walk through, but extremely painful seasons on top of it. Who would I be today had I not gone through these struggles? Where would I be today had I not fought hard everyday to pick myself up and keep going? My friend, your season of anxiety, isolation, pain, heart ache or whatever you're going through – you're not alone. Our struggles are the beautiful unseen sculptures in our lives molding us into who God has intended us to be. The scars we have aren't meant to keep us in shame, they're meant to remind us of the battles we've won, the victories we've conquered.

Whether you're struggling in the midst of a season of isolation, or another challenging circumstance, there is in fact light at the end of the tunnel. You may be fearful about how your life will be the same after going through this difficult time but let me remind you, this is the beginning of the next chapter of your life. You are a beautiful, worthy, courageous Joyful Warrior and your battle has already been won! This is not the end of your journey, these trials are not meant to break you – a season of growth and healing awaits! If you would like further accountability and a safe please to talk please email me at info@joywarriorbook.com. I would love to walk along side of you no matter what stage you are at in your journey! God bless.

Take Action Now!

1. Affirmations! Don't forget to love yourself; speak love into your life and that of your loved ones. Whether your affirmations are speaking scriptures aloud daily, or motivational quotes, the best way to maintain a healthy positive mindset and move away from losing yourself with anxiety in isolation is to constantly remind yourself that you believe in YOU. Look in the mirror and pour your heart out with words of encouragement that you got this!!

Hemp + CBD Knowledge Hub

I am incredibly excited to be an affiliate partner with W!NK the industry's first CBD for women, by women! I hope you will take the time to review the information below, and that you will gain a better understanding of the amazing benefits of incorporating CBD into your daily regimen. My hope is that all stigmas will be removed on your path to mind-body wellness. You will further explore how this industry is growing at a rapid pace, for good reason. As women, it is so important to take care of our minds and bodies so that we can better serve others. Always want to be mindful of the products you not only put in your body but on your body which is why I recommend W!NK as they have carefully crafted exceptional wellness products and skincare products! Below you will find informational slides and two blog links that give a more in-depth look into the industry as well as W!NK.

My Affiliate Code: WinkKeiana01

My Referral Website Link: http://lddy.no/gdf9

Blog Posts (Click Below):

Important Things About CBD

Mind + Body Renewal With CBD

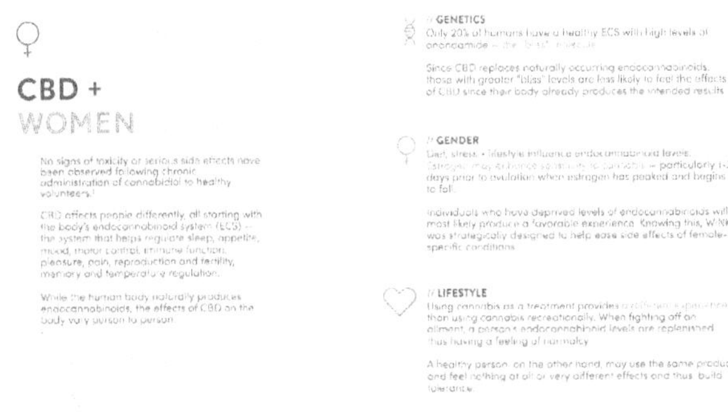

Photo Courtesy of W!NK

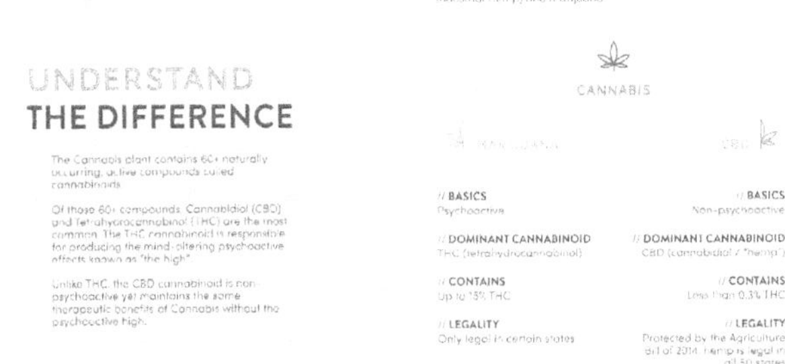

Photo Courtesy of W!NK

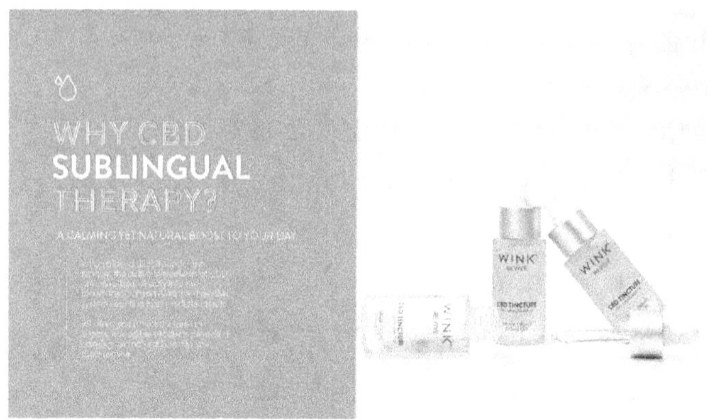

Photo Courtesy of W!NK

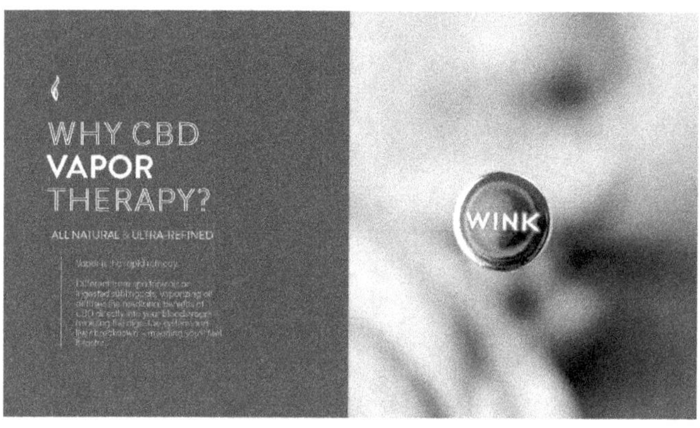

Photo Courtesy of W!NK

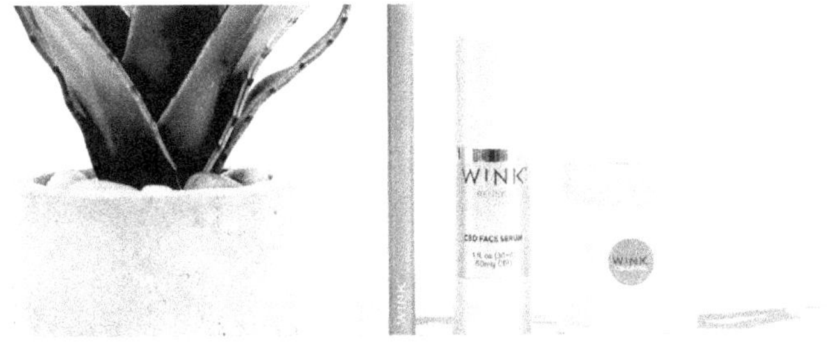

Photo Courtesy of W!NK

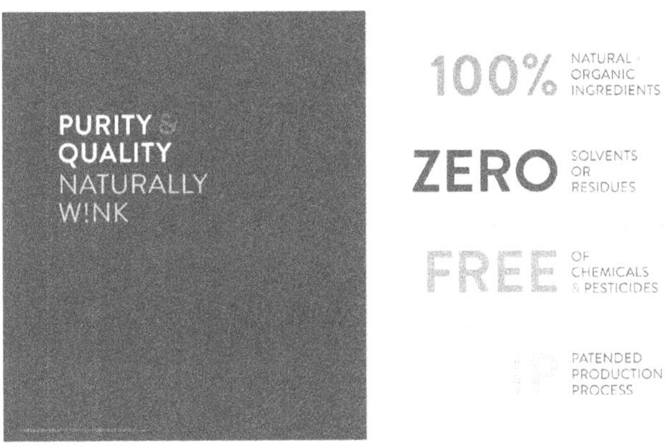

Photo Courtesy of W!NK

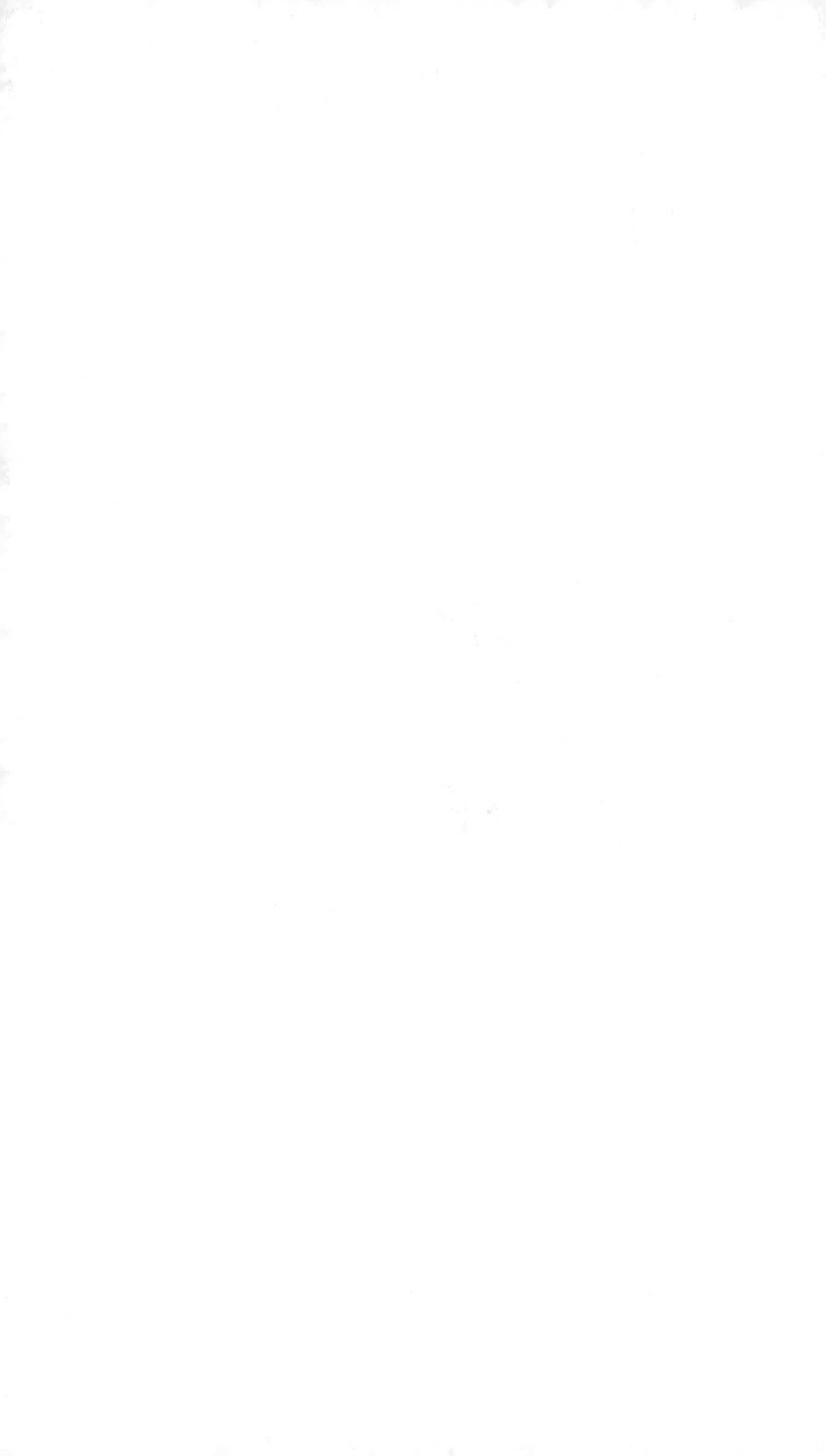

Warrior Directory

This directory is a resource I wanted to include to help guide you through some of my favorite products, apps (links for both iPhone and Androids will be included where applicable) and articles. I hope you'll find great use in some of these as you navigate through your journey as Joyful Warrior! *Note: Some of the links below are affiliate links and if you go through them to make a purchase I will earn a commission. Keep in mind that I link these companies and their products because of their quality and not because of the commission I receive from your purchases.*

Chapter 1
| Meditation Apps |
> *Abide*
https://apps.apple.com/us/app/abide-christian-meditation/id726031617
https://play.google.com/store/apps/details?id=is.abide&hl=en_US

> *Calm*
https://apps.apple.com/us/app/calm/id571800810
   https://play.google.com/store/apps/
details?id=com.calm.android&hl=en_US

> *Breethe*
https://apps.apple.com/us/app/breethe-meditation-
sleep/id920161006
   https://play.google.com/store/apps/
details?id=com.Meditation.app&hl=en_US

Chapter 2
| Gratitude Journal |

Journaling and/or gratitude journaling is an amazing way to let go. You don't need anything fancy, just a notebook and pen. I included here the app I use daily as well as a beautiful guided gratitude journal.

> *Day One*
https://apps.apple.com/us/app/day-one-journal/
id1044867788
   https://play.google.com/store/apps/
details?id=com.dayoneapp.dayone&hl=en_US

> *Erin Condren PetitePlanner Gratitude Journal*
https://www.erincondren.com/petiteplanner-
gratitude-journal-edition-2

| Lavender Oil |

> *Trinity Fit*

I love supporting women owned business. This is my sweet friend's company and I use not just this amazing lavender oil but all of her essential oils exclusively.

https://trinity-fit.com/keiana?wpam_id=2

Chapter 3

| Water Intake Tracking App |

> *My Water*

https://apps.apple.com/us/app/my-water-drink-reminder/id964748094

| Supplements |

> *Renova/True Hope*

This is one of my favorite companies as their products are centered around brain health. Their micronutrient supplement has over 20+ years of research in the area specifically on mental health. Please see the Research Summary of 34 publications on the EMPower Plus micronutrient supplement as well as link to purchase. I have been using this product for some time personally and has played a major role in helping my anxiety personally as well as a few of their other products.

https://worldvu.renovaworldwide.com/clients/
pandora/companycontent/policies/documents/
empowerplus_research_summary_2019.pdf
https://keiana.renovaworldwide.com/shop/

> *Juice+*

My beautiful friends are partnered with another great supplement company as well. If you're having trouble getting enough of a variety of fruits and veggies they have amazing 30 plants conveniently encapsulated to help bridge the gap. They have chewable for kids as well!

https://alexwoodworth.juiceplus.com/us/en/buy/
capsules/juice-plus-fruit-vegetable-berry-blend-
capsules

Acknowledgements

First and foremost I was to thank Jesus Christ, my Lord & Savior! Words can't truly express how humble and grateful I am for the opportunity to produce a piece of work to help others during a difficult time.

Thank you to my Graphic Designer: Claire is a creative artist residing in Long Beach, CA with her fiancé and their little dog. She makes a living as a freelance 3d artist supporting top brands at festivals and conventions. In her free time she enjoys supporting like-minded women as they create brands and build successful businesses. Collaborating with Claire has brought the look and feel of this important guide to life. I honestly don't know how this project would have come to life without all of your help Claire Bear!

Thank you to my Editor: Charvelle Holder-Dobard is a writer, actress, and plus size model living her dream in Los Angeles. With a degree in Journalism from Emerson College, she moved out west upon graduating, and hasn't looked back since. A *Jill of All Trades*, she generously agreed to copy edit this e-book and believes it to be an important resource for all. Your guidance and wisdom with this project made a path for me to fall so much more in love with writing. Thank you.

Thank you to Dr. Caroline Leaf, Rachel Hollis and Ed Mylett for inspiring me to become the best version of myself. For creating content that teaches me that I matter. Reminding me that chasing my dreams and striving for more in life is OKAY! We were all meant to do more in life.

As special thank you to all of my family and friends who have linked arms with me in one of the hardest seasons of my life; you know who you are. There are always going to be the highs and lows in life, I am so blessed to have certain people who uplift me, encourage me and continue to push me outside of my comfort zone. I love you all so much! xo

Thought Provoking Questions

1. If you could make one change today based on the information that you've learned from this book, what would you immediately implement to improve your quality of life?

2. What are you currently doing to help ease your mind that is currently working for you in your life?

3. In your isolation and/or your own personal hard season, where do you see yourself on the other side? What can you take away it?

Contact

For more information, wellness coaching or support
please visit my website:
www.manifoldstrength.com
Email: info@joyfulwarriorbook.com
Instagram: @manifoldstrength

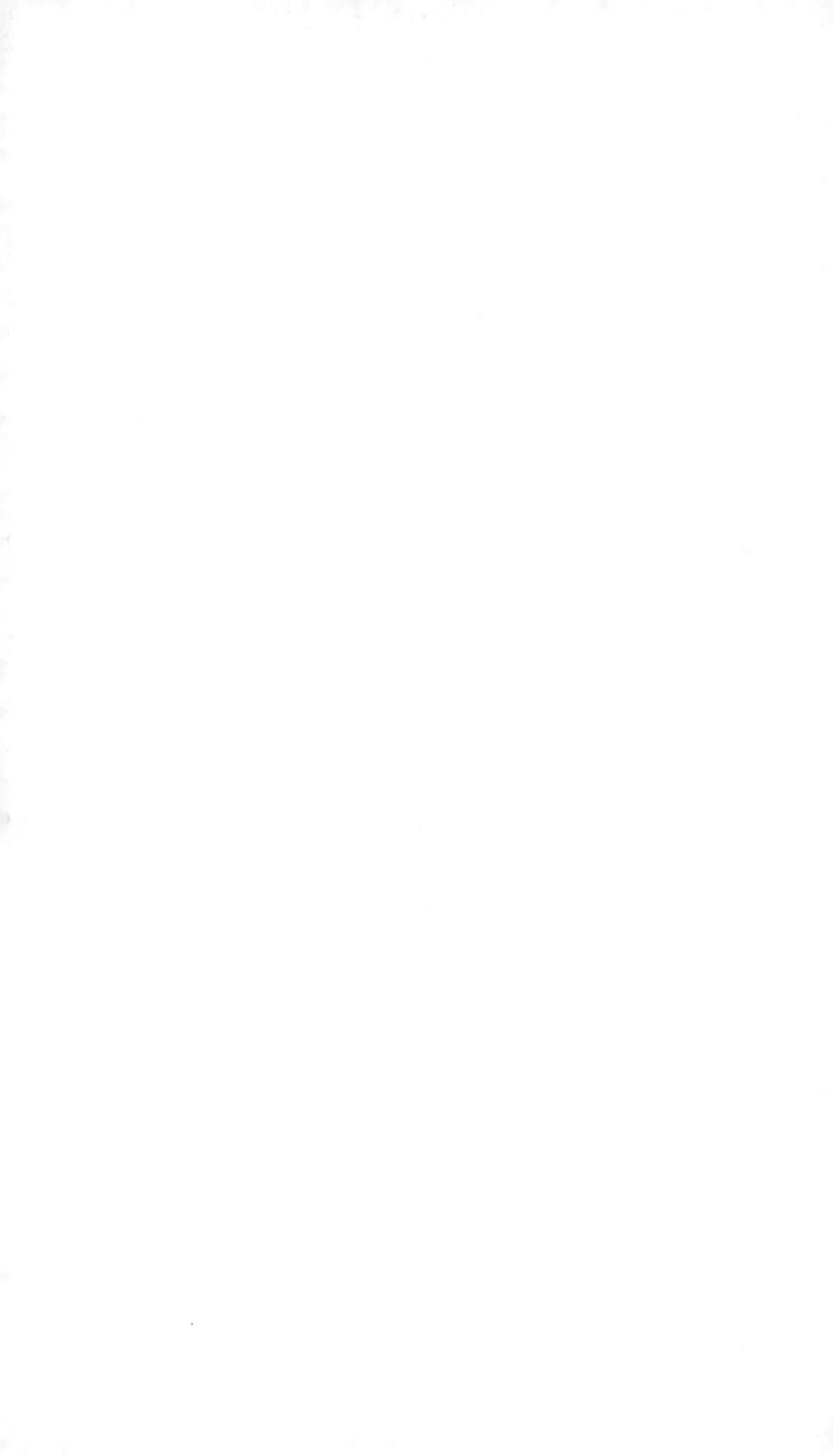